Front cover photograph. Children o.
Lane Estate, playing in the sand, d
tion of Anderson Shelters in 1940.

Best wishes
Anne Rogerson

SAFFRON'S HEALTH
DEPENDED ON WEALTH

A look at health care for residents of Saffron
Lane Estate before the National Health Service

Published by Coalville Publishing Company Ltd.

Typeset by Steve Duckworth at The Springboard Centre, Coalville.

Printed by Norwood Press.

ISBN 1 872479 13 8

Contents

FOREWORD

This book is a product of the Saffron Lane Estate. Without "The Saff" it would not exist. The project began almost eighteen months ago, born of an idea of the Women's Group which meets at Linwood Centre. They had just shared their experiences of modern-day health care, producing a booklet called, **"Don't ask us we're just the patients"**, when one of the group wondered,

> "But what must it have been like before the National Health Service?"

From such a simple question came this collection. I was fortunate enough to be appointed as Oral History Project Organiser and have worked with the Women's Group, and a wealth of other volunteers, devising questions, taping interviews and finally writing up our findings. All the people interviewed either live, or have lived, on the Saffron Lane Estate. The oldest contributor was born in 1903, whilst the youngest one is a mere 63 years old. For this reason the stories told refer to a period from about 1906 until the Health Service was started in 1948. Most of them though are really about the inter-war years from 1918 until 1939, but particularly from 1925, when people first came to live on the Saffron Lane Estate.

This book is not intended as a definitive history of health care before 1948, but it is, hopefully, going to bring back memories to those who lived through the period and give those who are too young to remember an insight into life at the time. For this reason I have included general historical information in the Introduction, for those who may want some more detail as background to the stories. I have not attributed the direct quotes from the tapes since some of our contributors wanted

1

to remain anonymous, a wish which we on the project must respect. For the benefit of those who cannot remember money before 1971, it is probably worth noting here that all financial figures quoted are from the period studied and therefore pre-decimal. There were twenty shillings (20/-) in a pound and twelve pennies (12d) in a shilling, or 240d to £1. That means one of our pence (1p) is equal to 2.4d. Enjoy the calculations as you read through!

We are grateful to all those who were so willing to give of their time and share their memories, so making this collection possible. I believe the results may best be summed up by one of the people who lived on The Saff from its earliest days until the 1950s:

> "These are my memories, the way I remember things as a kid, other people may have different ideas, but these are mine."

Enjoy the memories!

Anne Kendall Rogerson MA

September 1992

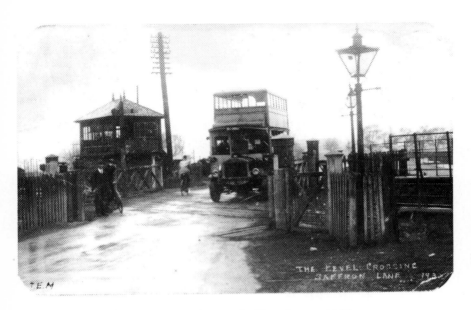

The level crossing at Saffron Lane, 1932.

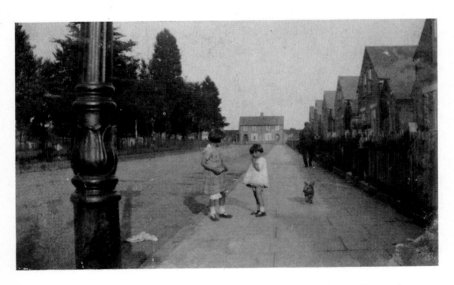

View down Copinger Road looking towards the railway line, about 1930.

INTRODUCTION

The National Health Service was introduced in 1948 based on principles set out in the Beveridge Report of 1942. It planned to provide for the citizens of this country comprehensive health care,

"From the cradle to the grave".

It was introduced by the Labour government which came to power in the landslide victory at the post-war general election of 1945. Before 1948, health care had largely been linked to the provisions of the National Health Insurance Act of 1911. Under this Act free medical care by general practitioners was available to those insured through work. It was often known as the "ninepence for fourpence" Act, since the worker (employee) paid 4d from the weekly wage, with the employer paying 3d and the state contributing 2d, to make up the total value of the 9d (ninepence) National Insurance stamp. This Act provided for some 15,803,000 insured persons between the ages of 16 years and 65 years whose incomes were below a specified minimum level. This was, at first, set at £3 per week but rose during the period so that in the mid 1930s it applied to all whose wages were below £5 per week, which was the majority of manual workers.

Those covered by the Act could choose a doctor and, subject to the doctor's consent, they would register on his/her list as panel patients. This medical benefit was administered by local Insurance Committees. However, the sickness, disablement and maternity benefits provided in the 1911 Act were administered by Approved Societies. Many such societies had long operated as Friendly Societies, which developed for the mutual support of their members, all of whom joined voluntarily. Amongst these Societies probably the best known are the Ancient Order of Foresters and the Oddfellows. The operation of the new Health Insurance Act was to be through Approved Societies, which meant that all who came under the provisions of the Act had to join a Society as a state (sometimes called NHI) member, if they wished to obtain benefit. Workers above the income limit also had the chance of joining the scheme as "voluntary contributors" by paying the full value of the National Insurance stamp into the Approved Society.

The criticism of the 1911 Act was that it only provided a general practitioner service and did not include dental, opthalmic (eyes) and hospital treatment or consultant services, unless by special arrangement (and usually at extra cost) with Approved Societies. It also failed to provide medical benefits for the dependants of insured persons. As a result, one alternative was for such dependants to become voluntary members of Approved Societies. Even assuming that such a financial burden could be taken on by the family, many such people would have been refused membership. The voluntary member, unlike a state member, had to be passed by a doctor as being in a fit state of health — many of them would not have been (see quote at end of chapter). A second course of action would have been for dependants to be insured in doctors' "clubs", which were run by general practitioners with fees of approximately 6d for adult, and 3d for child membership, which would be collected locally, usually each week. For those who could not afford either of these provisions there was no alternative but to pay the doctor's bill privately, which was usually out of the question, or rely on the outpatients departments of the hospitals.

It should be pointed out that rudimentary health care for school children up to the age of 14 was provided through the school clinics. The headquarters of that service in Leicester opened at Richmond House in January 1921. These facilities existed for the treatment of minor ailments, dental treatment and even the supply of spectacles, at rates according to the family income. The clinic also had facilities for carrying

5

out operations such as the removal of tonsils. There was a minor ailments and school dental clinic, which opened in 1928 and was based in the wooden structure in the grounds of Marriott Road School.

Many of the hospitals of the period are still in operation today, though their functions may have changed over time. Treatment at a fever hospital or a sanatorium would normally be provided at public expense. The sanatorium for the treatment of tuberculosis (TB) was a vital part of medical provision. TB was estimated to have been responsible for 15% of all deaths in the United Kingdom in 1918. It was felt that a cure would never be found for the scourge which hit rich and poor indiscriminately.

The two other major hospitals which served the area were the Leicester General Hospital, which began life as the North Evington Poor Law Infirmary in 1905, and the Leicester Royal Infirmary (LRI), founded as a voluntary hospital in 1771. The first rule relating to the admission of patients at LRI stated,

> "All persons unable to pay for adequate medical attention are admissible for relief in the Institution."

Historically the hospital was funded by donations from private benefactors and officially a patient should have been recommended by one of these benefactors (i.e. someone paying towards the financial support of the hospital) for treatment. Beds and cots were endowed, either in perpetuity or on an annual basis. Hospital Days were held which were carnivals where money would be collected to help in the running of the Infirmary. The Saturday Hospital Fund also raised money. In 1919 it levied subscriptions at 1d per week, but these were raised to 2d in 1920. For this subscribers were supporting not only the hospital, but also the convalescent homes, which meant members were entitled to a period of convalescence if necessary. In 1927 the LRI Annual Report stated,

> "A record total of £44,080.15s.4d was reached. The Board offer their congratulations to the Society (Fund) on the record figures. 255 new subscribing firms were added to membership during the year."

The subscriptions for the Fund were stopped out of employees' wages. By 1938 the subscription varied between 1d and 3d per week, but it was roughly 1d in every £1 of wages earned. In 1942 the Hospital Fund gave the Infirmary an income of £46,700, with £18,000 on account for the Casualty and X-ray Building Fund. That figure may possibly have been higher had it not been for the war.

Our project has centred on the Saffron Lane Estate, but when it was being built the Infirmary Board of Governors were concerned about the extra demands such new house-building would place upon hospital services. In 1925 the Council bought land on the south side of the town for the Saffron Lane Park Estate. There were to be over 600 houses built there. The Council tried to ensure an attractive plan, straight streets were rarely used and four different house types were designed using a variety of building techniques and materials. Such new house construction worried the LRI Governors, however, as these comments from the 1927 Annual Report show:

> "Whether the additional housing provision be by 'Council' houses or through building societies, or private enterprise, demands upon the hospital surely follow. Rents make substantial inroads on weekly earnings; building society payments absorb, for the time being, surplus income. In such economic circumstances the artisan in the 'Council' house and the worker who secures his house through other media, both seek admission to the voluntary hospital when acute sickness comes. It follows that from thousands of newly erected houses in Leicester and Leicestershire, added demands are made upon the county hospital."

A comment on the health of those moving into the new houses can probably best be left with one of our contributors who had this to say:

"The first tenants of these houses [on The Saff] came from the slum clearance areas of Leicester where they lived in atrocious conditions. Whole families lived in one room, sharing a toilet with three or four other families with a stand pipe in the yard. When they came to this estate their standard of health was virtually zero."

Given that as a starting point, along with the background of state provision such as it was, please read on and find out how, in their own words, the residents did cope.

HOME REMEDIES

**"When anything was wrong with you, the first
thing Mam always did was say,'You need a dose
of physic.'"**

One thing that most contributors agreed upon was that in
cases of illness home remedies would be tried first. A trip to
the chemist was expensive and a visit to the doctor would be
out of the financial question for many individuals who were
not panel patients. For this reason, most people remembered
the home "cures" which were used, some being more effective
than others!

The dose of physic referred to in the heading of this chapter
was commonly used, many folk believed a good "clear out" of
the bowels would cure any illness. This would usually mean
drinking a mixture of liquorice powder and water or sometimes it was mixed with chloridine, or for others Albion
tablets were taken but,

> "You were not allowed to swallow them, you had to crunch
> them and they were horrible."

If the complaint was constipation, rather than just being
generally unwell, syrup of figs, a dose of (Epsom) salts or
senna pods were each commonly used as laxatives. There
were, or course, more specific remedies in use especially for
colds, coughs, cuts and the more common ailments. A sore
throat would often be treated with a sweaty sock.

> "Years ago when we wore socks you changed 'em once a
> week and if your feet sweat they were really nice and ap-
> parently if you tied a sweaty sock round your neck that is
> supposed to cure a sore throat. I have been to bed once or
> twice with a sock round my neck."

A different approach, but a similar idea, was tying a "tar" rope round the neck, which would be worn all day and at night to cure the sore throat. Sometimes a "noggin" or lump of butter would be mixed with sugar or taken from a spoon to ease a sore throat, or another commonly used relief was a salt water gargle. One person remembers wearing a vapour bag tied round the neck.

> "It was like a lavender bag but it was solid, by the time the winter had gone it was getting smaller and smaller."

It was used to help protect against catching coughs and colds.

If such attempts at prevention did not work though, there were cures at hand. A cold would be treated by cutting up a lemon, pouring boiling water over it, leaving it to cool and then drinking the liquid. Soaking feet in a mustard bath was also reckoned to be a good remedy for a cold or a chill. If the cold settled on the chest, goose grease was used.

> "We used to have a goose at Christmas if we were lucky, then Mother would save the grease, put it in a jar. This goose grease would be rubbed all over your back and front to ease your chest and make you cough easier. Goose grease is like dripping you used to put it on brown paper and put it on your chest and back."

A similar treatment was applied using a tallow candle, instead of goose grease, to help a chesty cough. Rubbing in camphorated oil was another favourite remedy for a bad chest. The oil, which would usually be warmed on the old fire range, was rubbed in back and front at night time. However, many home remedies sought to use items readily to hand. Several people told us of being encouraged to go and smell the tar as the gangs worked on surfacing the roads — that was supposed to improve a bad chest and cost nothing.

Another remedy for coughs and colds was referred to as "hecky pecky" wine. Several contributors told us of its use for a chesty cough and one explained how it had been used

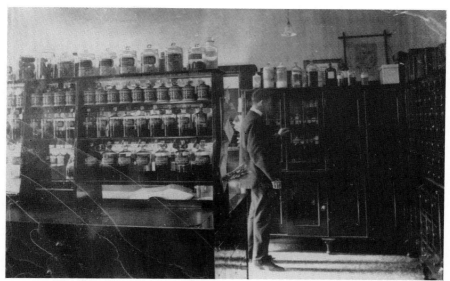
The Dispensary at Leicester Royal Infirmary about 1905.

George) only applied to persons over 16 years of age. There was, therefore, a two-year period between leaving elementary school at 14 years and becoming a panel patient at 16 years of age, where no state provision existed even for those in full-time employment.

Some doctors ran their own "clubs" which provided cover for medical expenses. Both Dr English and Dr Power ran such clubs, employing local people as collectors. The idea was that any member of the family not covered as a panel patient could have the services of a doctor in times of sickness. It is interesting to note that many of our interviewees were still not covered by medical insurance of any kind, simply because their families could not afford the contributions. However, some families did take up the offer of such cover. These were the memories of two sisters from the late 1920s:

> "My mother had to pay 3d a week for the children and 6d for herself. Our family was a bit exceptional because some of our neighbours were very poor. We weren't well off, but we weren't poor to some of 'em. One woman got turned

out because she couldn't pay her rent, although her husband had a job it didn't pay very much. But we could afford the doctor's club and I think it was Mrs Belton's daughter who used to come and collect it every week."

During the period we are looking at there were two doctors' surgeries which operated on Saffron Lane. Dr English had a surgery listed at 513, Saffron Lane, whilst Dr Power was at 519, Saffron Lane, both being near the City Arms public house, which has recently closed. Although Dr English owned the house in which his surgery was held, he had caretakers living there. His main surgery was at his own home on Aylestone Road. The surgery on Saffron Lane operated almost as a branch office. Dr Power lived on the premises and held surgery in a room within his own home. He also had a dispensary.

"The doctor used to make up the medicine while you waited."

Dr Power, however, left the area after being taken ill. One contributor told us this, although no one else mentioned it.

"I remember Dr Power was took ill and I think he had TB but when he got better he wasn't able to come back because he sold his house to Dr Freer."

(Information held at the Leicestershire Record Office shows Dr Power was practising in 1932, but the next available records show Dr L. Freer and his wife Dr Helen Freer were practising from that address by 1936. Owing to the "one hundred years closure" rule on medical records it was not possible to verify whether Dr Power did suffer from TB.)

Dr L. Freer and Dr Helen Freer were married and both were listed as general practitioners in 1936. Dr Helen Freer continued to work on the estate until well after the introduction of the National Health Service in 1948.

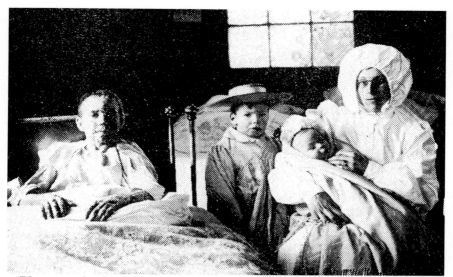

Photograph of Dr Maurice Millard as a two-year-old during the 1903 Leicester smallpox epidemic. The photograph was intended to show that recently vaccinated persons need not fear the disease.

Other doctors whose practices would cover the estate were Dr Morrick, with a surgery on the corner of Aylestone Road and Cavendish Road, Dr Millard at Grace Road, and Dr Snoad also of Aylestone Road, who used to visit his patients using a horse for transport.

Dr Maurice Millard was the son of Dr Killick Millard, who was Leicester Medical Officer of Health from 1901 until 1935. The photograph above shows Dr Maurice Millard, the older of the two children, at the bedside of a smallpox sufferer in the 1903 Leicester smallpox epidemic. His father arranged for the picture to be taken as a practical demonstration that recent vaccination gave complete immunity to the disease. It obviously did because the boy standing closest to the bed survived to become a well known local doctor.

A visit to the doctor's surgery was different from today. The one thing most people commented on was the absence of an appointments system. Many spoke of the advantage this had, namely of being able to see the doctor on the day you wanted to, but it did have a down side too, as this memory shows:

> "You used to have to wait a couple of hours or so to see the doctor in the surgery. You used to get there early if you could, but I have queued up out of the surgery, outside and down the passage. The passage wasn't covered in. I suppose the doctor started at a certain time and finished when the last person had gone. There was a morning and evening surgery."

The following description tells of a visit to the surgery of Dr English, who had caretakers living in the house.

> "Her front room was his surgery. When you went in you sat in her living room. All the while you were there she sat at the side of the fireplace. There was a row of chairs along the back wall and you dare not make a noise or speak. In the doctor's surgery itself there was a desk, a row of shelves and a couple of chairs, but I don't remember there being a couch or bed for examinations."

Sometimes people from Saffron Lane would go to Dr English's other surgery on Aylestone Road, but this memory suggests that it was rather different.

> "It was quite posh, there was carpet up there, but it was lino on the floor at Saffron Lane."

The same contributor spoke very highly of the treatment received from Dr English:

> "He was a very good family doctor. He would always come."

A contributor who was sharing her own memories of the late 1920s around Wharf Street in Leicester suggested that there was preferential treatment for "private", as opposed to panel, patients. Although she was later connected with the Saffron Lane estate these coments do not relate to any doctor who practised on The Saff.

"I remember going once and somebody saying, 'Oh the doctor's got a private patient', so the panel people had to wait while the doctor saw the private patient. I don't know if that happened all over, but it did near us. People getting a doctor's bill got priority. You would just sit and wait. You never talked to anyone in the surgery, the only time anybody moved was when they coughed. The first door was one surgery then there was the best surgery, that was for the private patients, we could use that sometimes, but mostly we used the first one."

If people needed a home visit a message would usually be sent to the doctor, either by word of mouth or by sending a child with a note, because telephones were virtually unheard of on the estate. Most interviewees who called the doctor spoke of them as being kind and helpful. It was interesting that no criticisms were made of the medical professionals. However, several people did comment on them as individuals. Dr Helen Freer seemed to excite most remarks, many referred to her,

"Always having a cigarette in her mouth"

and more than one commented on her long polished fingernails, but they seemed agreed that she was,

"Direct, to the point and a very good doctor".

Dr Snoad was also one whom people remembered as rather a character, telling of his home visits made by pony and trap.

Perhaps, though, the secret of the popularity of the doctors who practised on the estate was their concern for their patients. One contributor must deserve to summarise this:

"The doctor was very very good. I can remember him being lovely. There was someone in our street couldn't pay and he was ever so good to them. I will always remember that."

It must not be forgotten, though, that whilst individual doctors proved themselves to be sympathetic in cases of particular need, there was a whole body of people on the Saffron Lane Estate for whom no real access was available to general medical help, simply because they could not afford it. As one contributor neatly summed it up:

> "People who couldn't afford that [i.e. paying a doctor's bill or a weekly insurance] either went without a doctor and dropped down dead or took really ill and were taken to hospital."

For those who could see a doctor, the dispensary would be their next port of call. Dr Power dispensed his own prescriptions as already mentioned, but others would go to "Pegg's Dispensary". It was located on the estate on the corner of Fayrhurst Road and Marriott Road.

> "The family who lived at the house were called Pegg and they had two rooms downstairs. They hired out the front one to the dispenser, but they didn't have anything to do with the dispensing side of things. Lots of people went there. That was in the thirties."

There was a contributor who was a friend of the girl who lived at the house. She told us how the front room used to be locked up except when the dispenser was there.

> "We weren't supposed to go in that room."

A third memory of Pegg's Dispensary came from someone who remembers being sent there as a child.

> "The dispenser operated from the front room. He had a little bit cordoned off with a counter and bottles behind him. You queued in front of the counter. I remember coming out with a dark blue poison bottle. It must have been poison because all the poison bottles were blue. I could not have been more than 10 or 11 years old."

Hearts of Oak Benefit Society.

ESTABLISHED 1842.

REGISTERED UNDER FRIENDLY
SOCIETIES ACTS, 1896 — 1924.
Secretary :
   T. S. NEWMAN,
     Barrister at Law.
TELEPHONE: EUSTON 2411 (5 Lines)

APPROVED UNDER NATIONAL
HEALTH INSURANCE ACT.

In your reply
please quote
CET/HS
P.C.Dept.

Hearts of Oak Buildings,
Euston Road, London, N.W.1

8th March   40.
_____ *19* ___

Headed notepaper of a Friendly Society.

The contributor added that the idea of sending a child that age on such an errand today horrifies her, but nobody thought anything about it at the time. If people needed in-patient care or were too poor to afford a general practitioner they would attend the hospital, the subject of the next chapter.

HOSPITALS AND CONVALESCENT HOMES

"It was different then to what it is now, much more strict."

Several of our contributors had memories of hospitals. Some of them concerned the isolation hospital and the sanatorium, which are dealt with in the section on infectious diseases, but others related to the Leicester Royal Infirmary and the Leicester General Hospital. The Leicester Royal Infirmary was a voluntary hospital but the General Hospital was originally a Poor Law Hospital. (See Introduction for more information.)

For some there were vivid memories of a visit to the out-patients department, brought on by some childhood accident.

> "I went down there because I was playing on the ocean wave [a type of swing] and my leg got trapped underneath it. They looked at it, then put a cold compress on it and bandaged it up. I was pushed round in a pushchair for about a fortnight after that."

Sometimes, though, the accidents resulted in a stay in hospital, as this did:

> "I was chasing round the table and it had very sharp corners. I misjudged it and hit my eye on the corner, it literally scooped my eye out. My Dad had to carry me down to the Infirmary with my eye on my cheek. They kept me in for a week and thought I would go blind, but it didn't seem to affect my eye at all."

People usually made their own transport arrangements for getting the injured to hospital. One man told us that he was probably one of the first traffic casualties on the estate, when

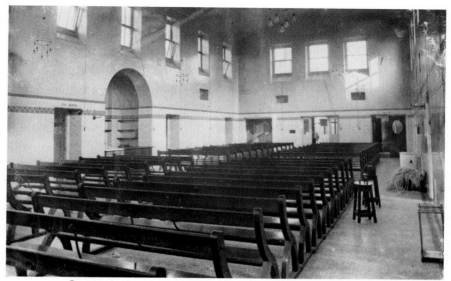

Outpatients waiting hall, Leicester Royal Infirmary.
Notice the pile of washed bandages on the floor waiting to be wound.
The bandage winding machine can be seen on the stool. Children
would often be asked to wind bandages whilst waiting.

he was knocked over by a builder's lorry. As a four-year-old with a $1/2$d in his hand he dashed across the road to the sweet shop and was knocked over. He was carried over the road to his house and was then,

> "Taken into hospital on my Father's crossbar. They said, 'You should be kept in', but for some reason they couldn't keep me in. Looking back on it I should have been, I was taken backwards and forwards on my Father's bike for treatment. I had fractured my skull. I can always remember at the top of Saffron Lane with the junction of Aylestone Road, just as you turn right was Freemans Common which used to be allotments. There was a small pub and on the side of this was the Mitchell and Butler's sign with a picture of a stag leaping over. I used to look to see this stag. I wasn't bothered about the treatment at the Infirmary, I was just fascinated by the picture of this stag leaping in the air."

It is difficult to know the reason why this child was not hospitalised in the late 1920s, but Rule 2 of the General Rules relating to admission to the Infirmary stated,

> "Patients who, in the opinion of the medical officers are capable of receiving equal benefit in the out-patients department, are not admissible as in-patients."

Many people were admitted, though, and hospital life in the 1920s through to the 1940s seemed strict when compared with today. At least two accounts told us of patients being strapped down to the bed. One in the early 1920s suffered from St Vitus' Dance.

> "I was strapped down at Leicester Royal Infirmary so I didn't dance about and hurt myself."

Another has memories from 1939 of a brother suffering great pain with kidney stones being,

> "Tied down with bedsheets",

at Leicester General Hospital. However, despite the strict way of running things, one patient of 1930 had this to say:

> "It was nice in hospital, they were very good to me. The nurses' uniforms were all starched, when they walked about you could hear them, you knew who was in the ward. The sisters had what they used to call bonnet strings. The matron was ever so strict. She used to come down every morning and look to see what the nurse was doing. The care was very good."

One contributor had memories of being in hospital with his brother. One of the nurses was taking a holiday in Blackpool and on her return brought a stick of rock as a present for each of the seventeen children in the ward! Another of our interviewees seemed to have a close knowledge of hospital life, he told us,

> "I kept them going down there."

At the age of 5 he had an acute appendicitis which was operated on, but later formed an abscess, so tubes were used to drain it. As a young child, he ran up the yard and crashed into his mother just as she was coming out of the kitchen door with a dolly tub filled with boiling water straight from the copper. It went all down his arm and shoulders.

"I was rushed down the Royal Infirmary by tram. Skin grafts were just coming in new, it was about 1915. I've still got the scars but when a doctor examined me in 1945 he asked if they were from the war and I told him when I had them done. He said I was very lucky because without them I would have had a crooked neck all my life."

Broken bones were another reason for a visit to the Infirmary. Not many contributors could remember having X-rays, although the hospital did have X-ray facilities at the time, but it was a relatively costly process. Splints were commonly used on broken arms. As one person told us,

"I was everlasting breaking my arms when I was a kid. They were forever on boards or splints, then they were bound up ever so tight, you couldn't move them, most uncomfortable. They were all strapped for weeks. You couldn't get dressed or undressed, things had to be cut and fastened round your neck. I seemed to spend half my childhood with my arm strapped in a bent position."

On being asked whether there was any physiotherapy available after the splints were removed, the reply was this,

"Oh no. The board is off, you're alright now."

Plaster casts were also used to set broken limbs. One person told us,

"A plaster cast would be put on by the local doctor sometimes."

Plaster of Paris was mixed with water and applied on a bandage over the limb which was then supported until it had set. Another remembered this though:

25

"If you broke a bone in your leg an iron was set into the plaster so you could still go to work because if you didn't work, you didn't eat."

One ailment which children may go into hospital for nowadays was not always dealt with in hospital in the period being studied. Several people recalled having tonsils removed at the school clinic. It would be done using a general anaesthetic, usually the ether mask. Sometimes the patient would only be kept for the day, as this man was in the early 1920s:

"I would be 7 or 8. It was like a school clinic at Richmond House. There was a dentist there and doctors were there. I went in at morning and came out in the afternoon. My sisters had to come down and take me home in a push-chair."

The Richmond House School Clinic opened in January 1921 and was on the corner of Richmond Street and Asylum Street.

A second contributor remembers having her tonsils removed at the school clinic during the 1930s, but she was kept in overnight. She recalled,

"Waking up and being very thirsty, so thirsty I could hardly speak. They wouldn't let me have a drink, just kept telling me it would make me sick. In the morning I woke up and there was a cup at the side of my locker. I drank the whole thing straight down, it tasted horrible. I later discovered it was senna tea."

(Senna tea was used as a laxative.)

The strictness of the regime in hospital extended to visiting times. Visitors had to queue outside the ward until the staff allowed them in. There were only two visitors per bed and visiting was strictly timed. It was usually from 3 pm to 4 pm on Wednesday, Saturday and sometimes Sunday afternoons. The food seemed to have been acceptable, if not exciting, though one man's abiding memory of hospital food was cabbage!

"I remember there was a lot of cabbage in hospital — it put me off cabbage for years."

One interviewee suggested the war caused a relaxation in the visiting rules.

"Through the war when servicemen were in you were allowed in every night for an hour then, but say there was something going off like the Padre or somebody went in to see them that was it. You didn't get in and we complained once and she [the nurse] said you can always come another night."

As a voluntary hospital, Leicester Royal Infirmary was keen to maintain its income and so was grateful for contributions made through the Saturday Hospital Fund. For the majority of people, starting work meant contributing to the Fund.

"You didn't have any choice you paid 1d for your Infirmary and 1d for your convalescent."

That memory comes from someone who started work in 1922 on a wage of 7/- per week, out of which 2d was paid to the Saturday Hospital Fund. That contribution then allowed the person who paid to go to a convalescent home if necessary, usually after an illness in hospital, but not always. Paying subscriptions to the Fund meant that individual workers were then technically contributing to the Infirmary. For historical reasons anyone treated there, because it was a voluntary hospital, should have been recommended by a person contributing to the hospital's finances (see Introduction). One of our interviewees told us the story of the panic which was felt in 1942 by her Mother because she did not have what was known locally as a "recommend".

"My Mother dare not go to keep her appointment because she did not have a recommend because they used to come and ask for them whilst you sat in the waiting room. I was working by then but my Father was too ill to work so he couldn't get one from where he'd been working. I went and asked where I worked. They gave me one but my Mum was ever so worried."

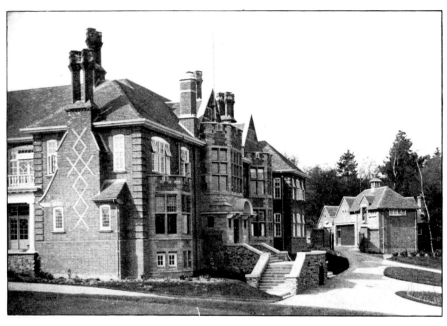

Swithland Convalescent Home about 1928.

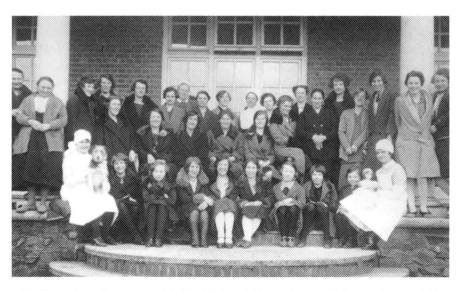

Staff and patients outside Swithland Convalescent Home about 1930.

The Saturday Hospital Fund at first ran three convalescent homes. They were Desford Hall for men, Swithland for women, and in 1919 a convalescent home was opened for children at Woodhouse Eaves. In 1932 the Saturday Hospital Fund moved its headquarters to Overstrand in Norfolk and in 1934 opened a home there for women, followed by one for men the next year. We learned this about the convalescent homes:

> "I remember going to Swithland, they took you up Mowmacre Hill in an ambulance. There was two of us, we were strapped to the stretchers but we had our feet against the door. I was terrified."

Once the journey was over, though, the interviewee was pleased by what she found.

> "It was really lovely, in the country and that. There were four of us in the ward. They learnt you to walk again and really looked after us. It was like a big mansion place and there were lovely grounds."

Another shared this memory:

> "I know my mother was pretty run down because she worked as well as keeping house. The doctor suggested she went to a convalescent home, so she went to Overstrand for a week on the Saturday Hospital Fund."

Someone else remembered going to Roecliffe Manor at the age of 11, which would have been in the early 1930s.

> "I went to Roecliffe Manor because Dad paid in to the convalescent home fund. I went for two weeks and I had never been away from home. We always had breathing exercises in the afternoon. Your parents were allowed to come and see you on the first Saturday after you got there."

The contributor suggested that the idea was to give the mother a break, because she had nursed the child through the illness and was probably in need of a rest herself. The

children were taken for outings to Bradgate Park and each
night they had to take a bath. The convalescent homes all
concentrated on providing fresh air and good food in an at-
tempt to build up their patients. All those who experienced
convalescent care spoke very highly of it. It should not be
forgotten that for the vast majority this would be a completely new experience since holidays away from home were almost unheard of for many families on The Saff at that time.
It must be remembered, though, that some people's hospital
experience would not have involved the Infirmary, the
General or the convalescent homes, but rather the
sanatorium or the fever hospital which were needed to deal
with the life threatening infectious diseases — the subject of
the next chapter.

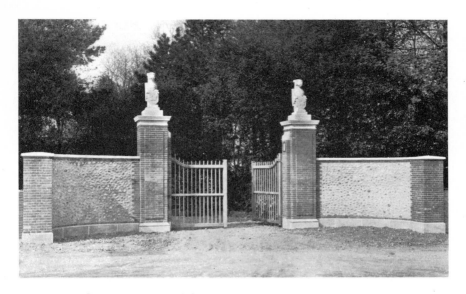

Overstrand Hall Convalescent Home entrance gates.

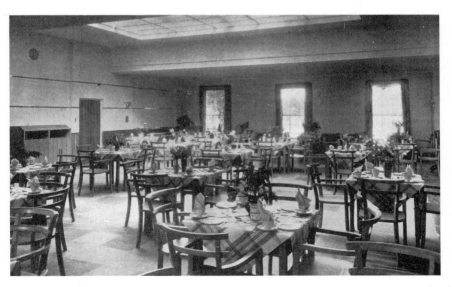

Dining room at Overstrand Hall.

INFECTIOUS DISEASES AND HOSPITALISATION

"There were three families in our street had TB and my Mam wouldn't let me have anything to do with them because it used to spread."

In the first half of this century people lived in fear of some particularly contagious diseases, which often proved to be killers. TB, scarlet fever and diphtheria were commonplace and difficult to cure. It is significant that almost without exception all our interviewees knew someone, or knew of someone, who had suffered from one of these infections.

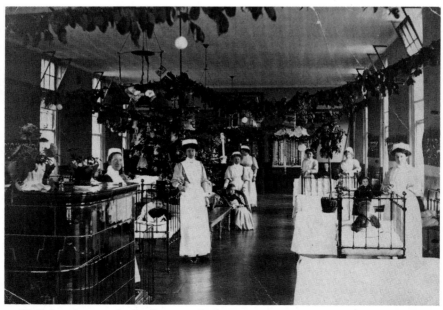

Children's ward, Groby Road Hospital around 1923, decorated for Christmas.

Diphtheria and scarlet fever usually meant treatment in the isolation hospital. For the city that was the Groby Road Hospital, which was also the sanatorium. The county had its own isolation hospitals, one of which was at Markfield. One of our contributors remembers having scarlet fever when she was about 6 or 7 years old, which would have been in the early 1930s. She told of being taken in a fever ambulance from Saffron Lane to Groby Road and that her Mother was not allowed to go with her, she said,

> "It was really scarey. When you got there the first thing they did was bath you, because I suppose a lot of children were dirty. I was at Groby Road for a start, maybe a week or so and then they took you to like a convalescent, what they called Anstey Lane, it was like wooden huts at the back."

She spent about three weeks there and throughout the whole time was kept isolated from her family, visitors could,

> "Just look through the windows at you."

Whilst she was in hospital the house was fumigated. She was told about it by the rest of her family at a later stage.

> "Mum said they did something in the house and put all sticking paper in it, so nobody could go in for so many hours, to try and get rid of the germs, but I was the only one who got it."

The routine was strict in hospital. She was kept in bed all the time and there was never any idea of toys being made available for the children to play with. Although she was isolated from her family and outside contacts, she was in a communal ward; there was no isolation within the hospital itself since all patients on that ward were suffering from the same disease. At the end of the isolation period people simply returned to the community.

"When I came out I know we had to walk a heck of a long
way to get on a bus, it seemed it anyway. Nobody had a
car and you couldn't afford a taxi so we had to walk to the
tramcars. When you came out there was no ambulance."

The idea of the isolation was the thing which most people
recalled,

"I can remember my Mum coming to visit me but she
couldn't come inside the door, so my Mum being worried
walked all round the hospital and got to the window so
she was standing on a basket on the outside. This nurse
saw her and went and pulled the basket out to let her feet
down. That was mean because you're not allowed to come
in at all."

However, some patients did not find the situation was too un-
happy. A third scarlet fever sufferer, in Groby Road during
the First World War, was asked her opinion of her stay there
and she summed it up in three short words,

"I loved it."

Diphtheria cases were also isolated from their families and
could expect to remain in hospital for about six weeks on
average. One person who went into hospital for a mastoid
operation on her ear caught diptheria whilst she was a
patient. She was then taken to Groby Road Hospital where
she had memories of talking through the window at the once
weekly visiting sessions. She has rather more vivid
memories of the general nursing though. She developed
scabs on her ears which she kept picking off, despite being
warned not to. In the end the nurses bound the card used
for temperature charts round her arms with bandages. In
this way both arms were completely stiff and she had no
choice but to lie there. They were only taken off at meal times
and then put on again. She remembered it stopped her picking her scabs though!

One interviewee was taken into hospital as a suspected "germ carrier" after her brother caught diphtheria. She was under observation for four weeks but received no treatment other than swabs being taken round her mouth. Her sister was also taken in as a potential "germ carrier" for the four weeks, but her brother was kept in hospital for twenty two weeks before he recovered.

However, the real killer disease of the period was TB. More than one contributor echoed the feelings of this one,

> "TB was spoken of as cancer is today."

The disease often began as a bad cold but continued to attack the lungs, the person suffering would usually lose weight and often die. There was no effective treatment until after the Second World War when new drug therapies were used with success. One woman summed up the hopelessness of the disease and its effect on the working classes in the 1920s with her story.

> "My sister-in-law lived with us in a four roomed house in Leicester. They took her to Markfield Hospital but they brought her home to me because she had no parents, so she came to me and my husband. They didn't give her hardly any treatment but she lived with us for about six months before she went back in to Markfield where she died, aged 21 years. It was worrying for me with having a baby but we couldn't do anything about it. In them days you had to go where you could, if we hadn't have had her it would have been the workhouse for her. We didn't get any screening ourselves — but it was very common, next door to me a father and son died within a fortnight of it. I was glad when we moved from that house on to Saffron Lane."

The treatment which was available was usually known as the "fresh air treatment". Patients went to the sanatorium which was usually Groby Road Hospital for people from

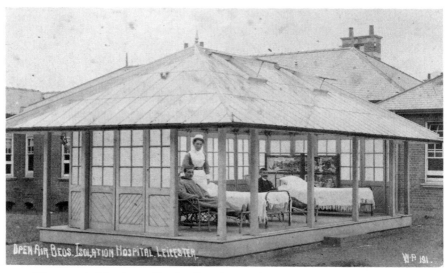

"Open air" beds at Groby Road Hospital Leicester about 1923.

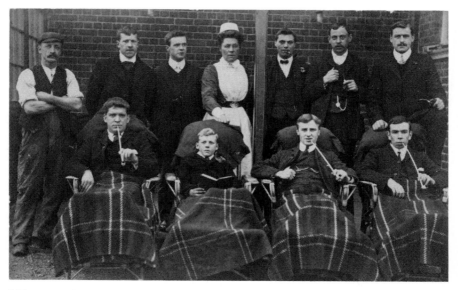

"Chest patients" enjoying their clay pipes at Groby Road Hospital about 1923.

Leicester. There the patients were put to bed on verandahs, open to all sorts of weather, to allow them to take the fresh air.

The photograph showing these beds dates from about 1923. The second photograph dates from the same period and shows "chest patients" enjoying a smoke from their clay pipes — a comment on medical opinion of the day perhaps!

There was no effective treatment for TB, or consumption as it was sometimes known, except for fresh air, good food and complete rest. It spread quickly through communities and several contributors told us of families where more than one member had died from the disease in a short space of time.

> "I remember one house in Marriott Road where three died in one family."

One sufferer who was first diagnosed in 1933 told us that,

> "They didn't compel you to go away [i.e. to the sanatorium] but so many obstacles were put in your way as regards work and anyway if you're that ill you can't work."

That particular patient spent seventeen years of his life trying to conquer TB. He underwent many experimental methods of treatment, including efforts to cause the lung to collapse. He was not cleared until 1951 with the use of strep-tomycin antibiotics. Someone else told us of his memories of a friend's mother who suffered from TB in the late 1920s,

> "She lived in a sort of wooden chalet in the garden. This chalet only had three sides and it was on rollers. The open side would be pushed round to face the sun. Her mother lived in that open-ended chalet all the time we were youngsters."

That was obviously not uncommon, for another contributor said,

"A school friend's father, who only used to do a little light work and then it would catch up with him, used to live in a sort of garden hut in the garden."

Despite the apparent difficulties of life in a sanatorium, one juvenile TB patient told us that admission to hospital meant it was the,

"First time I was fed right and had a good bellyful in my life, hospital was like being in a palace except people were dying all around — it affected you."

Children, as ever, saw things in slightly different terms. This person was admitted to a county sanatorium at Mowsley with suspected TB. He was there for sixteen weeks in 1928 and remembered fondly the community spirit which existed amongst children aged 8 to 16 years. They lived in huts on a swivel base, the whole end of which faced south and had huge doors, which were never to be closed. He recalled waking up with frost half way up the blankets on his bed. They lived next to nature, with a minimum of clothes on and received daily doses of a sun-ray lamp. They ate good food and were given regular liquorice powder medicine every weekend (see Home Remedies section). He remembered the matron ruling the place "with a rod of iron". Visiting was allowed once a week and he remembered,

"Mums and Dads always went away in tears, but we were happy as larks. We played and made huge snowmen, although we only wore plimsolls and shorts with no vests or socks. We seemed resistant to the cold. The sun-ray seemed to make us brown as berries too. The only thing was we didn't know who was going to die except that the ones who were going to die next were usually in bed."

Could this be why Mums and Dads usually went away in tears?

As there were so many killer diseases within society at the time, death appears to have been less of a taboo subject than it is today. When people died they were left in their own home until the time of the funeral.

"There was no such thing as going to a Chapel of Rest."

There would often be a local woman called upon to "lay out" the dead. One contributor explained how her mother was that woman for their area and that she herself once went along to help. This is the story she gave us:

"She would take the pillows away, lay the person flat, wash them and then tie up the jaws with a piece of bandage. The eyes would be closed then two pennies put on them to hold them down. The ankles would be tied together with a piece of ribbon, just until the person was really cold, then it could all be taken off."

After that the undertaker would be called to measure up for the coffin. It would be brought and stood on trestles in the front room for about three days until the funeral. The undertaker used to nail a black board or plank of wood on to the window so that all the neighbours would know there had been a death in the family. All the street would close their front curtains, some straight away, but everybody on the day of the funeral, as a mark of respect. Whenever a funeral went by people always stood still and,

"Every man would doff his cap."

One person explained that one of her earliest memories was of being allowed to look out at a passing funeral procession.

"We were allowed to look out with the curtains pulled tight round our faces so it didn't look as if they were open. There were six black horses with black plumes on the front of their harnesses and an old fashioned hearse. I can still remember the sound of the horses' hooves on the road as it went by. That would have been about 1930."

On the following pages, copies of bills for such a funeral can be seen. These bills relate to a brother and a sister. One died of TB and the other of meningitis. The parents had a third child, born a month after the second funeral. That child survived and kindly loaned us these documents. It is interesting to note the approximate three-fold increase in cost, for what seems to be similar provision, during that nine-year period. Such a funeral would be very expensive for a family on an average income of between £2 and £3 per week. It has been suggested that funeral expenses were often offset by insurances known as the "penny policies". Having considered death, it is probably appropriate to look at the other end of the life scale and discover memories of birth.

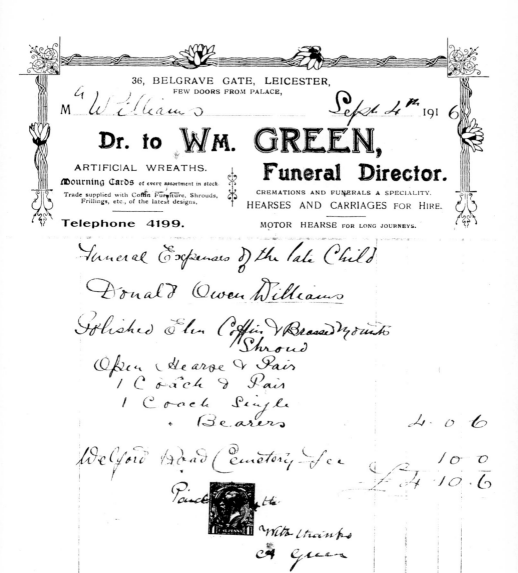

36, BELGRAVE GATE, LEICESTER,
FEW DOORS FROM PALACE,

M⁴ *Williams*   *Sept 4ᵗʰ* 191 6

Dr. to WM. GREEN,

ARTIFICIAL WREATHS.
Mourning Cards of every assortment in stock.
Trade supplied with Coffin Furniture, Shrouds,
Frillings, etc., of the latest designs,

Funeral Director.

CREMATIONS AND FUNERALS A SPECIALITY.
HEARSES AND CARRIAGES FOR HIRE.

Telephone 4199.   MOTOR HEARSE FOR LONG JOURNEYS.

Funeral Expenses of the late Child

Donald Owen Williams

Polished Elm Coffin & Brass Mounts
Shroud
Open Hearse & Pair
1 Coach & Pair
1 Coach Single
+ Bearers   4 . 0 6

Welford Road Cemetery fee   10 0
                                              £4 . 10 . 6

Funeral bill of 1916.

41

37a Belgrave Gate, also at
13 Montague Road, Clarendon Park, Leicester.

Feb. 6th 1925

Mr Williams

Dr. to John Newby & Son,

Funeral Undertakers.

Trade supplied with Coffins, Coffin Furniture, Shrouds, Frillings, etc.

Hearses, Carriages, and Motors for Hire.

Memorial Cards all Latest Designs.

Cremations and Funerals a Speciality.

Funeral Expenses of the late

Irene Ellen Williams

Polished Elm Coffin with Silvered Fittings
Swansdown Shroud
Open Hearse & Pair
1 Coach & Pair
1 Coach Single
Bearers   11 · 10 · 0
Purchase Grave for one Welford Road Cemetery
& Interment Fee   2 · 3 · 0
                                 £ 13 · 13 · 0

Settled with Thanks
Feb 6 1925

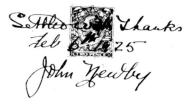

John Newby

Funeral bill of 1925.

BIRTH

"There weren't any preventions then, we never heard of it anyway."

Probably partly as a result of the above statement, made by one of our contributors who married in the 1920s, the birth rate was high and large families commonplace in the inter-war period.

"I had ten children, nine lived but one was stillborn."

Birth control methods were available but not easily and usually not free, so pregnancy and childbirth were a familiar pattern. One fact which was frequently reported was summed up by the person who told us,

"If you weren't married and had a baby then it was a dis-grace."

Most children were born at home, with the help of either a neighbour or a midwife. The neighbour would usually be an older woman who would be called upon in times of crises. She would be the one people would turn to for advice in ill-ness, help with childbirth and with laying out the dead. Most people made reference to one such woman they knew, but there were several, so obviously each operated within a small area of the estate. There did seem to be a general lack of knowledge.

"Sex was taboo",

and,

"Suddenly there was another baby there",

were fairly common remarks.

43

However, probably one comment which does sum up how little was known was that made in the early 1930s by a girl of about 13 years who went to school and told friends her aunty was going to have a baby. Imagine the poor girl's feelings when another girl replied,

> "It's not your aunty, it's your mother, she's got a big stomach."

Without doubt though, the heroines of the childbirth scene were Nurse Dodson and Nurse Green. The warmth with which people spoke of these two midwives was overwhelming. They were obviously about the best known and best loved characters of the estate. Both were listed as midwives in 1936 under the City of Leicester Midwives Act, but Nurse Dodson had certainly practised on the estate for several years before that. She originally lived on the estate in Windley Road and at that time used to go about her business on a push bike. Sometime during the early 1930s she moved to a house in Burnaston Road, near the City Arms, which she shared with Nurse Green. She later invested in an old Ford 8 car to get her around the estate, where she continued to work until the 1950s. Towards the end of her working life she suffered problems with her feet, and more than one person told us she often wore carpet slippers when doing her visits!

There did not seem to be much ante-natal care at the time we investigated. When a woman was aware that she was pregnant she would,

> "Book the nurse. She would feel round your tummy, check your water and that was it, not like they do now. It either came or it didn't."

The nurse would usually call at the mother's house shortly before the expected confinement to check all was ready for the birth, though many women worked virtually up to the birth. One person had memories of using "blocks to raise the bed up" to make it easier for the nurse. Giving birth was usually called confinement because it meant being confined to bed for fourteen days. Relatives or neighbours would usually take care of the other children in the family, since if the father had work it would be almost unheard of for him to take time off to look after the family while the mother was confined.

A local woman would often work alongside the midwife, being there with the mother when the midwife called, as she did usually every day of the fourteen-day confinement. The woman's role would be to make the mother comfortable and she would usually take any washing away and do that at her own home. Such women may or may not have been paid, but the midwife should have been. However, Nurse Dodson did not seem unduly bothered about her money! One interviewee suggested,

> "A good 50% of the estate owed Nurse Dodson money, but she never pressed for it, it [ie the job] was just the love of her life."

Another told us,

> "She was married but her husband had died in World War I so she took up midwifery. She never had any children of her own, but she must have brought thousands of babies into the world on Saffron Lane Estate — she was wonderful."

A third person paid this tribute,

> "She was ever so lovely and homely was Nurse Dodson. Both her and Nurse Green were very nice."

Sometimes the nurses would be paid in kind, with vegetables, eggs or flowers. One contributor told us the story of a teacher she was particularly fond of leaving school. She desperately wanted to give the teacher a present but had nothing to give and no money to buy anything. Nurse Dodson heard the story and promptly gave the girl some flowers she had been given that day for attending a confinement.

They then trimmed them up with some ribbon and the girl had a bouquet as a gift for her teacher, through Nurse Dodson's kindness. It was an act of kindness not forgotten almost sixty years later.

Most people could not remember the amount to be paid to the midwife, but one person had this to say:

> "When you had a confinement you had to pay a shilling a week until the midwife was paid. Then if you had a doctor you paid two guineas for him to attend the birth. The Foresters [see Introduction] didn't cover confinements, only ordinary medical things."

These memories were from someone whose first child was born in 1930. However, we are extremely grateful to one contributor who gave birth in 1947, the year before the National Health Service started and allowed us to copy the midwifery bill, which shows she had to pay £2 to Nurse Dodson for attending the confinement.

If a birth looked as though it may be complicated then a doctor was also called in. If the doctor was unable to resolve the problem at home then the patient was sent to hospital as was the case for this contributor in 1930:

> "I started labour at about 5 am but it was not easy. Three doctors came at home to try and turn the baby but couldn't. They took me in by ambulance down the Royal at about 11 pm, took me down to theatre at about 2 am then when I woke up I was in a side ward by myself. They told me the baby had passed away."

This contributor spent six weeks in hospital, for some of that she was "on the danger list" which meant her husband could visit her at any time. At the end of the six weeks she went

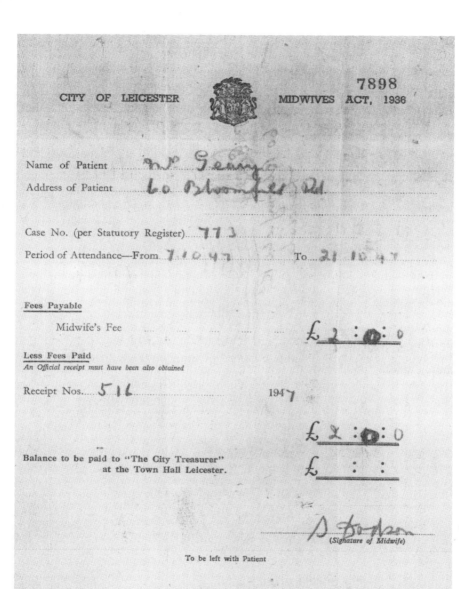

CITY OF LEICESTER   MIDWIVES ACT, 1936

7898

Name of Patient .... *Mrs Genny*

Address of Patient .... *60 Bloomfield Rd*

Case No. (per Statutory Register) *773*

Period of Attendance—From *7.10.47*   To *21.10.47*

Fees Payable

Midwife's Fee   ....   £ *2 : 0 : 0*

Less Fees Paid
An Official receipt must have been also obtained

Receipt Nos. *5 16*   194*7*

£ *2 : 0 : 0*

Balance to be paid to "The City Treasurer"
at the Town Hall Leicester.

£   :   :

....
(Signature of Midwife)

To be left with Patient

Bill for attendance of midwife at a confinement, October 1947.

47

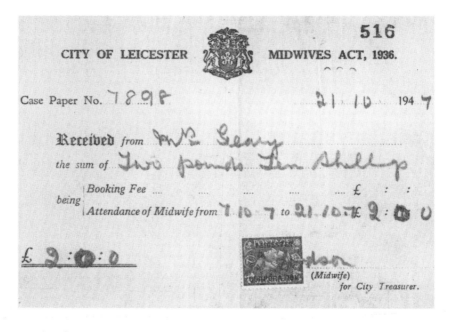

Receipt for payment of midwife for attending a confinement in October 1947.

for three weeks to Swithland Convalescent Home. She was not given any advice about future pregnancies, all the follow up available was,

> "They just told me I had to go back in six months' time to see if everything had gone back properly, but that was as far as it went."

She gave birth to a healthy child three years later at the end of an uncomplicated pregnancy. She also remembered,

> "Most people didn't go to the doctor's, it was only complicated cases. It was optional to go to the doctor's, it was only people that could pay, when you went to book you paid your money."

Although most people had babies at home, some did choose to go into hospital to give birth.

> "I don't believe in births at home. I felt better in hospital. There were six beds for confinement where I was in the City General in 1933."

One contributor chose to go into Bond Street for her confinement for which she remembered paying £3 in 1932. Another memory involved being strapped up with a bolster case and,

> "Having to lie on your tummy for an hour a day in bed whilst being confined."

However, not all was plain sailing. One woman remembered being booked into the City General in 1939 because things were not going well during the pregnancy but,

> "During my waiting time I had notice to say could I find other accommodation to have my baby because they were taking all the wards for the service people [1939 was the outbreak of World War II]. That was a very big shock to us because I wasn't having to pay to go in the City General, they didn't try to help me to get anywhere. In the end, I got into a little private nursing home in the Highfields. It

cost £8 a week and I was in for a fortnight. That was a lot of money because my husband was in the shoe trade, which was very bad."

Once a baby had been born, there was nothing in the way of special care baby units for small or premature babies, though one contributor had vivid memories of how Nurse Dodson and Nurse Green dealt with the problem.

"If the midwife had a tiny baby that obviously needed a lot of care and the mum perhaps had a big family or wasn't capable of coping with a very tiny baby she actually brought the baby home to her own home and she made a huge coal fire in her living room. She had a wicker linen basket and put a four folded big woollen blanket into it and then put the baby into it. Of course there were no draughts because it went right over the sides of the basket to keep it really warm. I can't remember what they fed it on but they sat up and took it in turns to sit up all night. I know because they asked me if I wanted to see this really tiny baby which was less then two pounds. I know it happened at least twice, one of the babies died but the other survived."

Miscarriage was not something about which much evidence came to light except one contributor who shared her own experience:

"I was seven months pregnant and I fell down when I was going to work and went on to my tummy but it took time to pull myself up. I still went to work that day — I worked in the shoes. But then I was bad and lost the baby. I was in City General for twelve weeks but I got a good constitution and pulled through. Twelve months later I had a baby with lovely golden auburn hair."

Perhaps it was that so many of these people had "a good constitution" or maybe it was the care of such dedicated community midwives, but despite the obvious hardships which many suffered there was little condemnation of the system from any of the contributors.

50

SCOURGES OF THE DAY

"My Mam used to wash our hair in vinegar to stop us getting nits."

Pneumonia, scabies, impetigo and nits were all common problems in the period we are looking at. Pneumonia was often a killer until after the Second World War, when drugs were developed to fight it successfully. Before that, there was no definite cure and no real treatment, other than good nursing care whilst the infection ran its course. Various reliefs were tried, such as linseed poultices which were used to stimulate the blood supply to the chest wall and so relieve the breathing.

One contributor told us that one of her earliest memories from the late 1920s was of having pneumonia and the care her mother took of her.

> "Where we lived everything was more or less in the kitchen, the copper, cooker, iron range, so it was a big kitchen and the stairs went up across the kitchen, not the stairs themselves, but the drop. Mum had a chaise longue under the stairs and she pinned a sheet from this stairboard to the other side of the kitchen where there were two shelves. The cooker almost came underneath this thing. She filled the old-fashioned kettle with the big spout and then made these funnels out of paper which she then shoved into the spout of the kettle and they were left to boil. The steam would come out of this funnel under this like a tent to help me breathe."

It was quite interesting that this person not only survived but also had experience of nursing a young relative through pneumonia, almost twenty years later, in 1947.

"The baths in the kitchen had a board top so that when you wanted a bath you lifted them up and hooked it, when it was down you used it for anything. We made him a bed on top of that bath, we got him a mattress down so we wouldn't have to move him from room to room, nobody could have a bath for weeks. We took it in turns to sit up with him. It was the night I sat up with him that they said this could be the night of the crisis, it will either make or break him. In the crisis, the temperature would go sky high. It did, he couldn't breathe and sweat was pouring down the poor little mite's face, he wasn't very old. I kept bathing his head and face with cooled water and all of a sudden he started to breathe and it got better until next morning he was a lot better. He still had pneumonia but he was over the crisis."

Theirs was quite an unusual family to have two survive, for many lost the battle against pneumonia. Another infection for which no real cure existed was tetanus. One account recalls a memory of someone in Marriott Road, in the late 1920s, who was very ill but he was not taken to hospital, probably because there was no cure or possibly because any movement would have caused the patient to go into spasm. Spasms happened after movement, loud noises or other disturbances.

"There were very few cars about then, probably the doctor was about the only one who could afford a car. The milk, bread and coal were all brought by horse and cart and they made quite a rumbling noise on the road so to keep it all quiet, whole bales of straw were opened up and put down in the road outside his house to deaden the noise. He later died. I don't think they got over tetanus in those days."

Not life threatening, but still unpleasant were the skin diseases of impetigo and scabies. Impetigo sufferers were painted with a purplish-blue liquid, called gentian violet. Everyone immediately knew, therefore, if you had impetigo. Many contributors told us of remembering friends who had to go to the school clinic and have the scabs pulled off, before being painted with the purplish-blue liquid, apparently a painful process.

Scabies was another skin disease, commonly regarded as a scourge of the times. One interviewee told how their family caught it as a result of her mother doing someone a favour. Her mother took in some washing for a neighbour and some two or three weeks later, first her father began itching, then her mother, followed by each of the children. It was diagnosed as scabies, probably caught from the dirty washing of the other family.

"My Mam cried, she was so ashamed, but the treatment really sticks in my mind. In Greyfriars there was a room and it was like a cellar and you had to go down steps and twice a week for weeks we had to go for these sulphur baths. There were two or three women in rubber aprons worked there. We had to go in turn into the bath and one of these women would come with a scrubbing brush and scrub your skin until it was sore. The sulphur was in the bath. We cried, but we had to do it, the whole family had to go. Most of our clothes were burned. There was a cubicle for each bath but I shall never forget having to be scrubbed, it was horrible, I was about 12 or 13 years old. The horror of those baths has stuck with me through all these years."

That same contributor went on to describe how a beautifully dressed woman and her young daughter who had both picked up scabies came in once whilst she was there having her treatment.

"She was obviously rich, she had a fur coat and everything but she was crying. I will always remember one of the women in the aprons saying to her, 'Don't cry — this thing breeds in cleanliness as well as in dirtiness.'"

Another common problem of the period was head lice. Most contributors had memories of the "nit nurse" coming to school.

"She lifted the hair up and gave a note to take home to those who had them."

Many mothers checked their own families for head lice.

"Mam would get a plain piece of white paper or a sheet of newspaper. You had to bend your head down and she would go through it with a fine toothcomb and the lice would fall out. The nits had to be picked off each hair or washed out with Derbac soap. That was a special black soap."

Some felt acutely the "shame" of having head lice. One contributor remembered this visit of the "nit nurse" in the early 1930s.

"When she came round, if anyone had got nits they were always pushed on one side, 'Go and stand over there.' Anyway, she came to me and she told me to go and stand over there, I was amazed. She then got this piece of paper and a steel comb and combed my hair. She got a little handful of nits, put them in an envelope and sealed it down. She wrote on the envelope, 'For the attention of Mrs _____ '. When I got home, my Mam couldn't believe it. I went through hell, she put this special stuff on my hair every night and used a steel comb. I was that ashamed that I went down to the clinic myself and asked the nurse to examine my hair before she next went into school. The nurse said, 'That's very commendable of you,' and she was pleased, but I just didn't want the shame of being dragged out of class again."

DENTISTRY AND EYE CARE

**"I remember my Grandfather had false teeth
and they were a dirty mulberry brown colour
not the colour of gums like they are today."**

Dental care and eye care did not appear to be high priorities
of life on The Saff in the period we investigated. Children
would have their teeth inspected by the school dentist who
operated from the wooden huts at the back of Marriott Road
School and from Richmond House. If parents sent a letter
stating that they had a private dentist, the children would
not have the school dentist attend to their teeth. This may
have been fortunate according to one description we heard
of practice at the school clinic in the early 1930s, this was one
ten year old boy's memory:

> "He pulled out two teeth, they had no injections or any-
> thing like that but they had a hook, put some cotton wool
> on it and put it in a jar that looked like iodine. Cocaine I
> think it was. They pierced it into your gum. When they
> pulled it out they wobbled it about. It looked like a bomb
> crater did your gum when he'd finished, nothing like
> today. It scared the life out of you and you never wanted
> to go dentist again."

The school clinics were keen to encourage people to go to the
dentist, though, as this interviewee remembers:

> "If you were good they used to give you a little tube of
> toothpaste, that was the school clinic at Richmond House."

Adults would have to pay for dental treatment and this would
partly account for why,

> "We never knew what a check up was."

One man recalled attending the dentist in 1932 when it cost 1/- for an extraction, but 1/6d for a filling. At that time he remembers earning 12/6d for a 48 hour working week, so dentistry was quite expensive in relative terms. People claimed they only went to the dentist when they,

"Couldn't stand it any more."

The equipment available to the dentist was very different then. People recalled the "hand cranked drills" so perhaps for reasons of cost and the equipment used, people preferred to have teeth removed rather than filled.

Any dental hygiene cost money, though many people did speak of having toothbrushes which they commonly used with salt.

"We didn't have a lot, so Dad used to say, 'Use salt with a toothbrush', we couldn't buy all the stuff you do today."

Others told of the old recommendation to,

"Put the brush up the chimney, that'll make your teeth white."

In other words, clean your teeth with soot. There obviously were products, such as toothpaste, to be bought for those who could afford them. One contributor, who was very proud of having had beautiful white teeth, said she used to be known as,

"The girl with the Solidox Smile",

in reference to an advert for toothpaste. Gibbs Dentifrice was the other brand name remembered.

Eventually, if people had lost all their teeth they may have considered having a set of false ones, others though just managed without teeth. One contributor told how his Father had a set of dentures made and the dentist had given him such confidence in the strength of these new teeth that he decided to put them to the test by placing them in the hearth and hitting them with a hammer — fortunately they passed the test! The dentures had cost £3 and that was more than a week's wages at the time.

However, not all the tales we heard condemned the dentists of the day. One contributor explained how she had been "larking about" at the age of 17 and knocked out part of a front tooth. She had the stump removed and one false tooth in its place, which was held in by a series of wires. She believed the wires led to the damage of several other teeth so that she needed more teeth removing. By the time her first child was born when she was in her early 20s, all her teeth had been removed and in 1932 she acquired a set of false teeth from Mr Hodges, a dentist in Belgrave.

> "I kept those teeth all those years until two years ago when I was getting a lot of ulcers and I went to the dentist on Aylestone Road and he said, 'My word you've had these a few years.' I got him to clean them and sort them out for me and I'm still wearing them and they're lovely."

In terms of eye care few people had memories of visiting an optician. Not many children wore glasses and those who did seemed conspicuous, were often teased and called names such as four eyes. One contributor told how she had always had bad eyes so at the age of five, she had her ears pierced:

> "The doctor did them and it cost 5/- and the sleepers were 7/6d which was a lot of money and I've still got mine. My Mam had to really save. They said if you had your ears pierced in them times it was good for your eyes."

She did not comment on what effect the ear piercing had on her eyes.

Glasses for school children were available and they were to be had free of charge if they were "school glasses from near West Bridge in Leicester" but many reported they were "horrible with steel frames".

Another contributor recalled,

"Most had tin glasses from down Carts Lane, but if you had tortoise shell you were posh."

The main source of optical help seemed to be Woolworths. Many contributors told stories of going into Woolworths and just trying on glasses until a suitable pair was found. The last word on eye care though must go to this interviewee. His comments sum up what was evident right through the project, that so many of the people who lived through difficult times; where money bought what we today think of as basic care and lack of money meant doing without; managed to keep their sense of humour.

"You used to go to Woolworths and they sold glasses of various strengths and they had a board there. You would try on different specs and when you could finally read what was on the board that was it, they were your glasses. I always said the reason they stopped that was there were so many people walking out with cheap glasses on and getting run over with the buses."

CONCLUSION

Thank you for reading this collection of memories. I hope it has given you as much to think about when reading it, as we had when researching it. The impression we have is that life was hard on The Saff for many of its residents, but that a combination of a sense of humour, determination and a developing community spirit pulled people through. That community spirit was summed up by this contributor:

"The neighbours when I was a kid were fantastic. They'd lend and borrow, beg but never steal, they were good as gold."

I think that sense of community spirit has been handed down. This project has come from some of the present-day residents of the Saffron Lane Estate. They have thought about it, researched it and criticised it as it has come to publication. They have worked as a team and any profit made from the sale of this book is to be ploughed back into Linwood Centre for use in that same community, so continuing the tradition.

On a personal note I would like to thank all those involved with the project for welcoming me into that community. However, I would also like to make a special mention of my parents, Charlie and Kath Kendall, who gave me the love, support and opportunity of the education which has enabled me to write this account. A final personal thanks to my husband, Simon, and daughter, Jemma, who encouraged me in this project and smiled through the chaos at home whilst the book was being written.

Anne Rogerson

AFTERWORD

We in the Women's Group believe that as our title says, health did depend on wealth for residents of the Saffron Lane Estate before the National Health Service was started in 1948. That is still the case for many of us today. Eye checks are no longer freely available, we know lots of people who do not go to the dentist now because they cannot afford to pay for the check up. Pregnancy testing is not always done by the GP, but it is possible to have a free test at Linwood Centre. Prescriptions are expensive, they cost £3.75 each and exemptions are not easy to get. We know about one sixteen-year-old who has a long-term medical problem and needs four different prescriptions every week. She has just started work and earns £50 a week, out of that she has to pay £15 for medicine.

The surgery on Saffron Lane has just applied for planning permission to extend so that more services could be offered there. At the moment there is no room big enough to offer ante-natal classes or similar meetings to do with health. The permission was refused because it did not include enough parking spaces. We thought this was a shame because most people using the surgery live within walking distance and many patients do not have a car in any case.

A lot of medical services have been centralised which means going either to the Infirmary or the General for help or treatment. It may not seem much to some people, but it costs money in bus fares to get to these places. We think it is worth making the point that money still does affect health care for people on The Saff today. It is not as bad as it was before the NHS because everybody can get to see a doctor without paying, but money is still an issue in the health of our community today.

Linwood Women's Group

Members

Dawn Bown
Jan Headley
Pam Kelb
Bernie Toon
Hazel Williamson

ACKNOWLEDGEMENTS

We on the project would like to thank all those who have helped in any way with the production of this book. This includes companies which donated the tape recorders used in the interviews, individuals who generously allowed us to use their photographs and documents, and the Leicestershire Record Office staff who have been helpful throughout the research phase of this project. Leicestershire County Council must also be thanked for their support of this venture, as must the staff at Linwood Centre. The sound technicians who copied and edited the tapes, along with the typists who processed the manuscript were all vital cogs in the wheel and we are grateful for their efforts. However, the main debt of gratitude must go to the volunteer interviewers and especially to the interviewees, for without them there would be no book. The names below include many of those who have helped, though it is by no means a comprehensive list. As stated in the Foreword, several contributors did not wish to be identified by name, but our thanks nonetheless go to them.

Jan Anderson

Peggy Briers

Jean Burbidge

Arthur Chimes

Eileen Chimes

Comet, Fosse Park

Dr W.J. Creagh

Rosamund Davies

Eastwoods Electric Superstore

Marie Geary

Carl Harrison, County Archivist
Margo Kirby
Jane Lawton
Leicester Mercury
Leicestershire County Council
Leicestershire Record Office
Bernard Lyner
Mavis Merrick
Thomas Merrick
Lydia Moreton
Kaye Nunn
Ruth O'Hora
Steve Peace
Les Price
Angela Reynolds
Jack Russell, Ancient Order of Foresters
Ethel May Sanders
Cyril Wood, Panasonic UK Ltd

BIBLIOGRAPHY

The following list represents books and papers used for background research and may prove of interest to those wishing to investigate issues raised in more detail.

Kelly's Directory of Leicester and Rutland, 1928, 1932, 1936 and 1938

Kelly's Directory of Leicester, 1951

Leicester Royal Infirmary Board of Governors Annual Reports, 1927 and 1942

Frizelle, E.R., Martin, J.D., The Leicester Royal Infirmary 1771 to 1971, Leicester No. 1 Hospital Management Committee, 1971

Webster, C., Health Services since the War, Vol 1, HMSO, 1988

Hodgkinson, R.G., The Origins of the National Health Service, Wellcome Historical Medical Library, 1967

Parry, N., McNair, D. (eds), The Fitness of the Nation: Physical and Health Education in the Nineteenth and Twentieth Centuries, History of Education Society, 1983

Stevens, R., Medical Practice in Modern England, Yale University Press, 1966

Hill, T.W., The Health of England, Jonathan Cape, 1933

Gemmill, P.F., Britain's Search for Health, University of Pennsylvania Press, 1960

Webster, C., Health, Welfare and Unemployment during the Depression, Past and Present, Vol 109, 1985

Do you remember Hospital Saturdays?, Mainstream, 9th November 1984

Cooper, W.G., The Ancient Order of Foresters Friendly Society: 150 Years, Executive Council of the Ancient Order of Foresters Friendly Society, 1984

Cunnington, C., A Brief History of the Leicester District, AOF, 1927

Minutes of the Committee of Management and the Investment Committee, AOF, 11th July to 12th December 1914

Rules of court "Heart of Oak" No. 3209, AOF, 1959

Willbond, W., A Home of Our Own, Leicester City Council, 1991